Preface

This manual is designed to be a guide to those who want to learn more about professional massage therapy. This is not meant to be a strict textbook of massage therapy or medical knowledge but rather it is a sample of what might be taught me a professional massage therapy instructor teaching a state specific certification course.

Please remember, that many states license and certify massage therapy. Before embarking on training or massage therapy for pay, please check with your state for specific licensing and training requirements.

The Television School of Massage Therapy was founded to give everyone more knowledge about the healing art of touch. Please visit our website for new and exciting product offers.

With the purchase of this manual, we offer a $3.00 off coupon toward the purchase of any of our products.

Release of Liability

The massage therapy techniques describes on our website, videotape, CD-ROM, DVD, and manual are for informational purposes only and are not designed to be an instructional guide for those seeking to be massage therapists. By viewing our website, videotape, CD-ROM, DVD, or manual the Viewer hereby voluntarily releases, discharges, waives and relinquishes the Television School of Massage Therapy (a.k.a. www.mymassagevideo.com), its owner(s), officers, agents, employees, independent contractors, business partners and volunteers, from any and all rights, claims, demands, causes of action and damages the Viewer now or in the future may have of any kind, now existent or which become existent in the future, whether the same be now known or unknown, and whether the same be now anticipated or unanticipated, resulting from personal injuries, death or property damage occurring to the Viewer as a result of participating in activities viewed or read on our website, videotape, CD-ROM, DVD, or manual and any activity(s) incidental thereto whenever and wherever the same may occur, and the Viewer does for himself/herself, his/her heirs, assigns, executors and administrators expressly **assume the risk** of such injury and/or death. The Viewer agrees that under no circumstances will he/she or his/her heirs, assigns, executors and/or administrators, present any claim for personal injury, property damage or wrongful death against the Television School of Massage Therapy (a.k.a. www.mymassagevideo.com), its owner(s), officers, agents, employees, independent contractors, business partners and volunteers based on non-willful conduct.

The Viewer, for him or herself, his or her heirs, executors, administrators and assigns, agrees that in the event any claim for my personal injuries, property damage and/or wrongful death, and/or any cross-complaint for indemnity and/or contribution arising there from, shall be prosecuted against the Television School of Massage Therapy, or any other person or entity released herein, caused by their non-willful conduct, including negligence, due to or arising out of participation in the activities set forth above and/or related activities that the Viewer will fully defend, indemnify and hold harmless said parties released herein from any and all such claims, judgments and causes of action by whomever and wherever made.

The Viewer acknowledges that he/she has read the foregoing two paragraphs prior to viewing or reading, is aware of and hereby assumes all of the potential dangers involved in or incidental to engaging in massage therapy, including, but not limited to the risk of injury or death.

Getting Started

Basic Necessities
- MASSAGE TABLE (cost: $150 and up)
  - Select proper height to reduce therapist strain
  - Chose portable or permanent style
  - Most are wood but some companies offer aluminum frame
  - Thickness of cushion/vinyl covering on table (for comfort)
  - Other options: Table, bed, floor.
- LINENS
  - Sheets (fitted twin sheets work best for most tables)
  - Towels
  - Pillows w/cases
- OILS AND LOTIONS
  - Many oils work good (base oil)
  - Almond, unscented coconut
  - Sesame, sunflower, safflower, etc.
  - You can scented oils
  - Colognes perfume, etc.
  - Essential herb oils (aromatherapy)
    - These are added to base massage oils
    - Some relax, de-stress, stimulate
  - Regular pre-made massage lotion most often used and can come scented
  - Talcum or other types of powders are used occasionally when oil isn't desired
- MISC
  - Music
  - Fan
  - Heater
  - Proper lighting

Selling yourself for success
- Business or greeting cards
- Gift certificates
- Discount packages
- Coupons
- Advertise

- Newspaper
- Radio
- Flyers
- Community service
- Trade for services
- If you haven't already, get more training
  - Anatomy
  - Physiology
  - Advanced massage
  - Stress
  - Yoga

MASSAGE ETIQUETTE

Health Benefits
- Helps blood pressure
- Increases circulation
- Helps to remove waste products
  - Drinking water in conjunction with massage helps eliminate toxin buildup thru urinary tract
- Promotes healing
- Helps joints flexibility and increases range of motion
- Helps the immune system
- Promotes better sleep
- It feels good…Don't underestimate the power of touch

Cautions of Massage
- People with recent operations or injuries (when in doubt refer to a doctor)
- Elderly people (varicose veins, osteoporosis.)
- Cancer, A.I.D.S., Leukemia
- Open wounds, rashes, acne, burns, etc.
- Fever

Helpful hints for a good massage environment
- Slow, relaxing, mellow music
- Access to a rest room
- Proper lighting
- Temperate conditions
- Quiet
- Clean
- Be Professional

Cautions of Massage

If you seek to be a professional massage therapist, check with state and local governments for specific requirements. In addition make sure you are covered with liability insurance just in case something does go wrong.

Specific Cautions
- Heart conditions
- Recent operations
- Varicose veins
- Cancer, leukemia, A.I.D.S., etc.
- Unused muscles
- Elderly people in general
- Pregnancy
- Open wounds, rashes, bums, acne
- Nerve damage
- Fever
- People on some types of medication

NOTE: Always get medical information. When in doubt, refer to a physician.

Massage Therapist's "Kit"

- Massage table
- Linens (sheets, towels, etc.)
- Oils (at least 2 types, 1 unscented)
- Music (slow, mellow, relaxing)
- Access to rest room (alcohol to sterilize hands)
- Accessories (hair clips, rubber bands)
- Business cards, brochures
- Room considerations
  - Temperature should be set for the client's comfort
  - Space should be enough for you to move around
  - Lighting is recommended to be low
  - Colors should be soft and soothing
  - Noise and outside distractions should be minimized
- Liability insurance: Make sure they tell you any important medical info, and sign a paper freeing you from any liability
- Get advanced education. Massage school-anatomy, physiology
- Be professional and make the client comfortable

Massage Etiquette

- Get the client to relax.
    - Let their breathing relax
    - Explain to them what you are doing
    - Address their need for modesty
        - Clothing attire for the client
        - Draping
        - Privacy
- Avoid "Compromising Situations" If someone makes an improper advance, it is up to you to not let it go any further
- Start client "face down" to establish a level of trust
- Avoid breaking contact, when possible
- Work towards heart, when possible to enable good circulation
- Be flexible
    - Change the massage from client to client, depending on need
    - Avoid "assembly line" massage
- Pressure
    - The deeper you go, the slower you go
- Keep a "safe zone" between your hands and groin area and breasts

Screening Clients

- Referrals-ask "How did you hear about us?"
    - Referrals show where you get your best business
- Ask:
    - "Have you had a massage before?
    - Do you have a particular problem (back, shoulders, etc.) you would like worked on?
    - Are you seeing a doctor?
    - Chiropractor?
    - Have you had surgery?
    - Are you on medication?" The client's medical background is very important
- Work out a payment plan that is comfortable for both of you. Note: Visa and MasterCard machines are available to anyone. Credit card companies take a percentage of what you earn from it. It may increase clientele about 20-30%
- Gift certificates are good tools. So are gift packages. Example: 4 one-hour massages for $100.00. You get your money quickly, and the client saves $5.00 a massage.

Benefits Of Massage

- Increases circulation
- Can reduce blood pressure
- Removes waste products (lactic acid, calcium, potassium)
    - Note: Drink extra water within 48 hours of the massage
- Makes muscles and tendons more flexible
- Speeds up healing process
    - Carpal tunnel injuries-preventative maintenance helps regression
- Reduces stress and tension
- Joints more flexible
- Decreases scar tissue by breaking up adhesions under the skin
- Reduces headaches
- Detoxifies the body quicker
- Promotes sleep and reduces tossing and turning
- Stimulates the body's immune system
- Can increase athletic or physical performance

Aroma Therapy

Definition:

- Use of essential oils (plant hormone extracts), added to massage oil to enhance the massage.

Examples:

- Eucalyptus soothes sore muscles, opens sinus
- Lavender relaxes
- Geranium eases stress
- Peppermint stimulates and opens sinus
- Camphor soothes sore muscles
- Jasmine relaxes

History:

- Developed circa 1900 by a French chemist, R.M. Gatte Fosse
- First known for antiseptic and antibiotic properties
- Herbs originally used were oregano, cinnamon, and clove

Aroma Therapy

- An aroma therapy distillation still consists of:
    - Vat: a large cylindrical tank, which contains the plants Steam is sent through the plants from the bottom of the vat and evaporates the oils.
    - Collection lid: A special lid, which collects the steam and sends it to the coil, usually refrigerated with running water, where the steam is condensed. The mixture of condensed water and oil separates naturally.

- Essential oils have hundreds of chemical components, most of them in very small amounts. No synthetic reconstruction can fully replicate a natural product Most qualified aroma therapists consider it essential to use natural essential oils.

Anatomy - Bones and Joints

Bones:
- Shapes of bones
  - Long (humerus)
  - Short (carpals)
  - Flat (ribs)
  - Irregular (vert)
- 206 bones total in body

Numbering system for vertebrae: (see diagram of full spine and vertebrae)
- Cervical = C1-7
- Thoracic = T1 -12
- Lumbar = L1 -5
- Sacrum = S1-5 (fused)
- Coccyx = C1-4 (fused)

Shoulder Girdle (see shoulder girdle shown on the skeletal diagram) (part of axial skeleton):
- Scapula (2)
- Clavicle ribs (2 pair)

Pelvic Girdle (see pelvic girdle shown on the skeletal diagram)
- Part of appendicular skeleton consisting of
  - Ilium
  - Ishium
  - Pubis
- Most bones when broken, take approximately 6 weeks to heal
- When massaging the back we can feel the spinous process of the vertebrae
- Ribs attach to the transverse process of vertebrae
- Seven cervical vertebrae are relatively small, and have holes (foramina) in their transverse processes
- Twelve thoracic vertebrae articulate with the twelve pairs of ribs
- Five lumbar vertebrae are massive, weight-bearing structures with limited mobility
- Sacrum consists of five
- Fused, modified vertebrae, and articulates with the two ilium bones to complete the pelvic ring
- Coccyx or tailbone is a vestigial structure consisting of three or four fused vertebral remnants

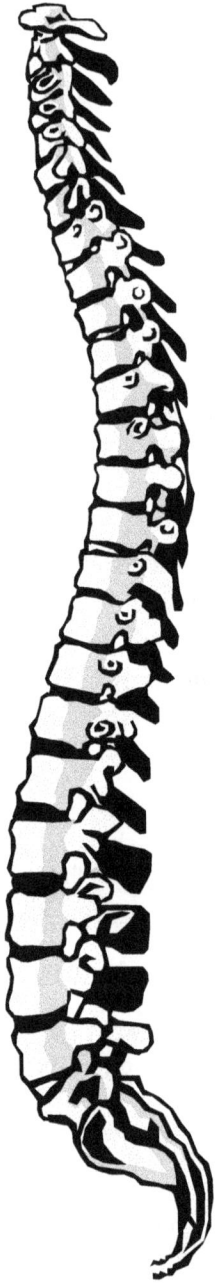

C1
C2
C3
C4
C5
C6
C7
T1
T2
T3
T4
T5
T6
T7
T8
T9
T10
T11
T12
L1
L2
L3
L4
L5

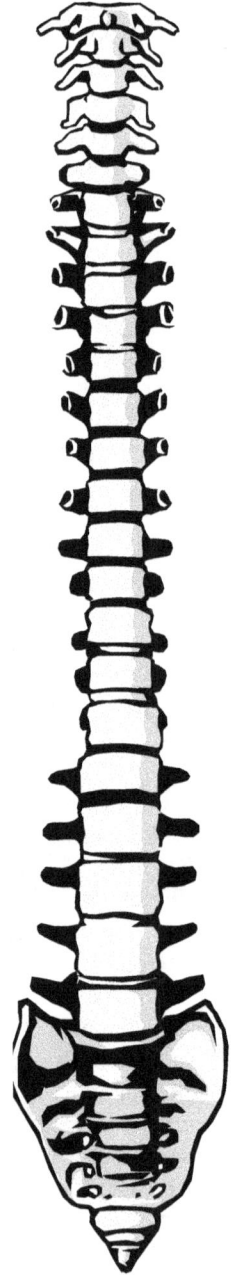

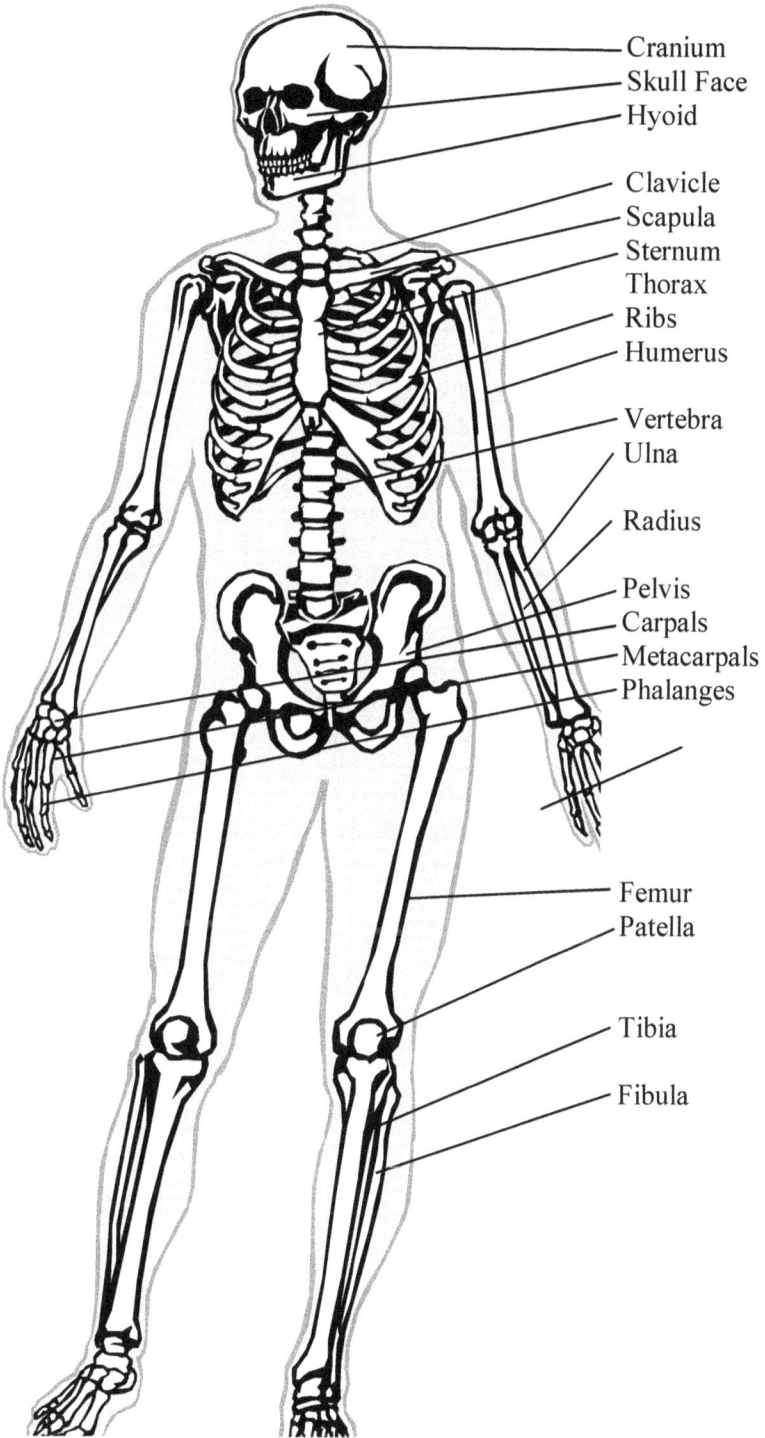

Cranium
Skull Face
Hyoid

Clavicle
Scapula
Sternum
Thorax
Ribs
Humerus

Vertebra
Ulna

Radius

Pelvis
Carpals
Metacarpals
Phalanges

Femur
Patella

Tibia

Fibula

Arthritis
- Inflammation of tissues surrounding a joint
- Drying and cracking of tissue is painful
- Loss of synovial fluid which lubricates joint

Osteoporosis
- A general weakening of bones. Often found in elderly
- Bones get weak and brittle

Osteosclerosis
- Abnormal bone growth (extra)

- Growth lines (similar to rings in a tree trunk), are found in soft spongy bones, are called episeal lines
- Atlas is another name for C1/Axis = C2
- Mother cells which make new bone cells are called osteoblasts
- We receive vitamin D from the sun (it helps make bones grow and heal)
- Bone is a living, growing tissue (It repairs itself, though an interconnecting network of blood vessels and nerves)
- Red blood cells made = soft spongy bone (ends)
- White Blood Cells made = Medullary cavity (2/3 made here, 1/3 made in lymph nodes)
- Periosteum is a fibrous connective tissue that covers bone. (Muscle tendon attaches to this)
- All bones are originally made from cartilage
- Sutures are expansion lines between sections of skull
- A microscopic look at hard compact bone, shows that it is like a honeycomb design
- Discs are like shock absorbers between each vertebra (made of cartilage).
- Bones not connected to other bones: Hyoid (front of neck) and patella (knee cap)

Each hand has 27 bones
- 8 carpals
- 5 Metacarpals are in your palm
- 14 Finger and thumb bones are phalanges

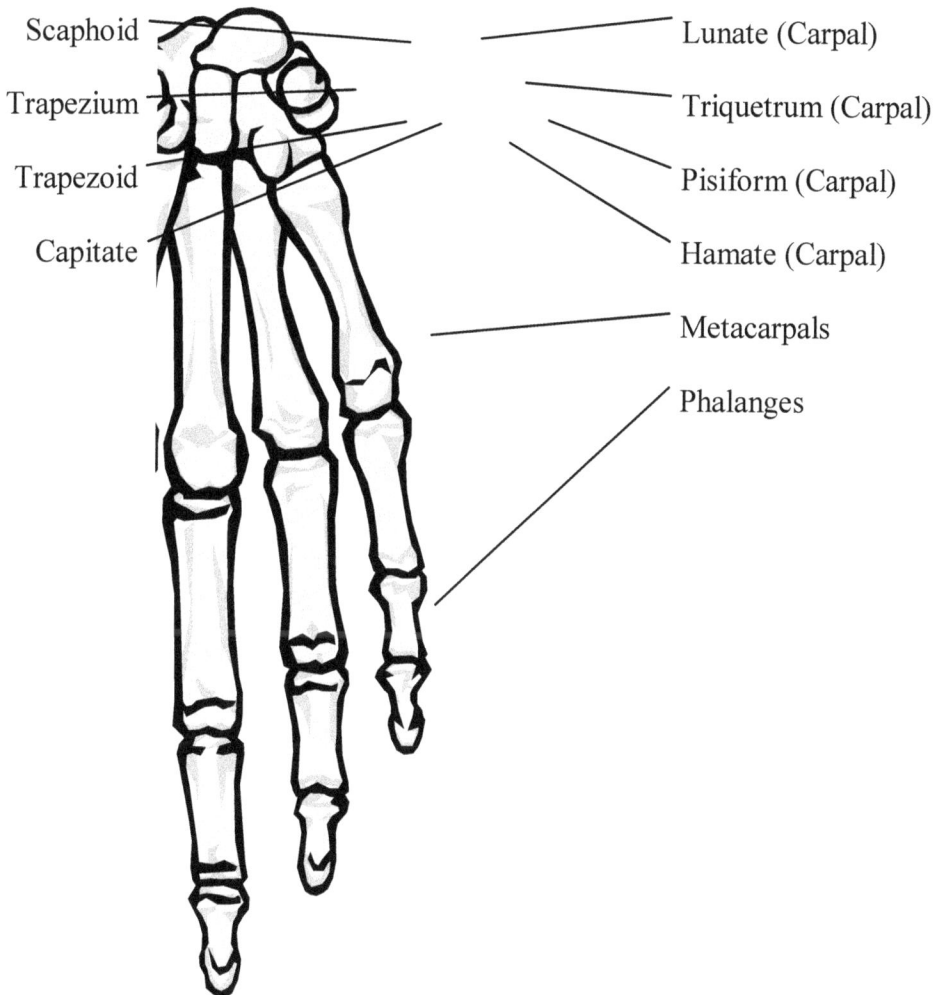

Scaphoid

Trapezium

Trapezoid

Capitate

Lunate (Carpal)

Triquetrum (Carpal)

Pisiform (Carpal)

Hamate (Carpal)

Metacarpals

Phalanges

Feet
- 7 Tarsals
- 15 Metatarsals
- 14 Phalanges

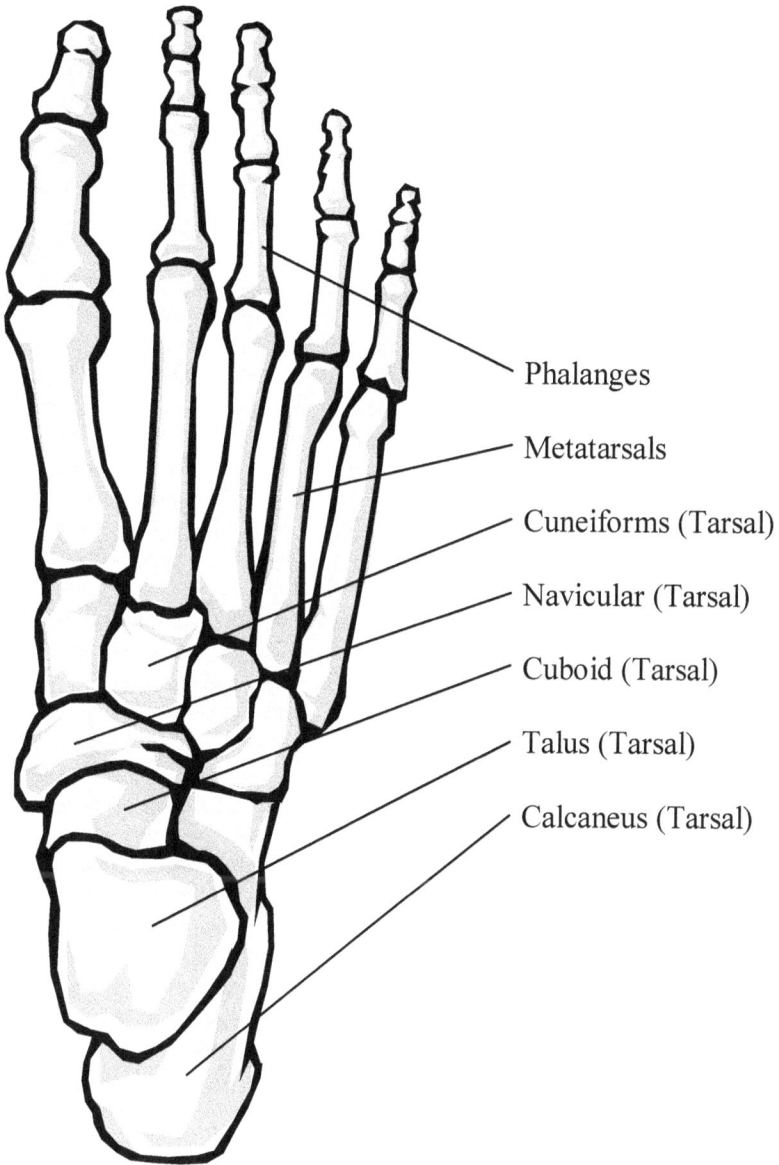

Phalanges

Metatarsals

Cuneiforms (Tarsal)

Navicular (Tarsal)

Cuboid (Tarsal)

Talus (Tarsal)

Calcaneus (Tarsal)

Knee:
- Patella
- Femur
- Tibia

Elbow:
- Radius
- Ulna
- Humerus

Hip and Shoulder:
- Illium
- Femur
- Humerus
- Scapula

Anatomy - Ligaments

Ligaments
- For support and protection of joints.
- Not very vascular (not much blood flow, so not many nutrients get to it).
- Contains many nerves making injury painful
- Not very flexible
- Requires long healing time

Anatomy - Skeletal System

- Axial
- Appendicular
- Humerus
- Radius
- Ulna
- Femur
- Tibia
- Fibula
- Carpals
- Tarsals
- Cranium
- Vertebrae
- Sternum
- Ribs
- Sacrum
- Coccyx
- Pelvis

Bone consists of:
- Spongy
- Medullar Cavity
- Compact
- Periosteum

- SKULL

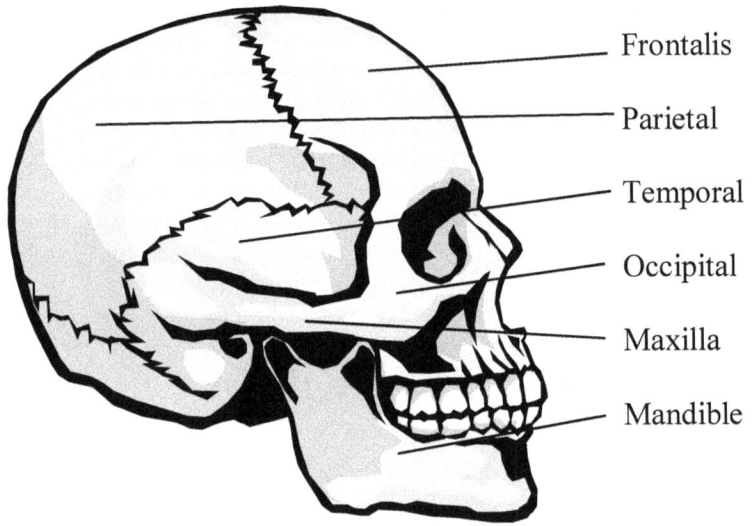

Frontalis

Parietal

Temporal

Occipital

Maxilla

Mandible

Vertebrae and spine
- Spinous process
- Transverse process (ribs attach here)
- Body
- Cervical (7)
- Thoracic (12)
- Lumbar (5)
- Sacrum (5)
- Coccyx (4)

- See diagram of vertebrae and spine in earlier portion of manual

Sacrum and pelvis
- Sacrum
- Ilium
- Pubic
- Ischium
- Coccyx
- Front view

- See diagram of pelvis, ribs and sternum

Ribs and sternum
- True
- False
- Floating
- Sternum
- Xiphoid process

- Diagram of pelvis

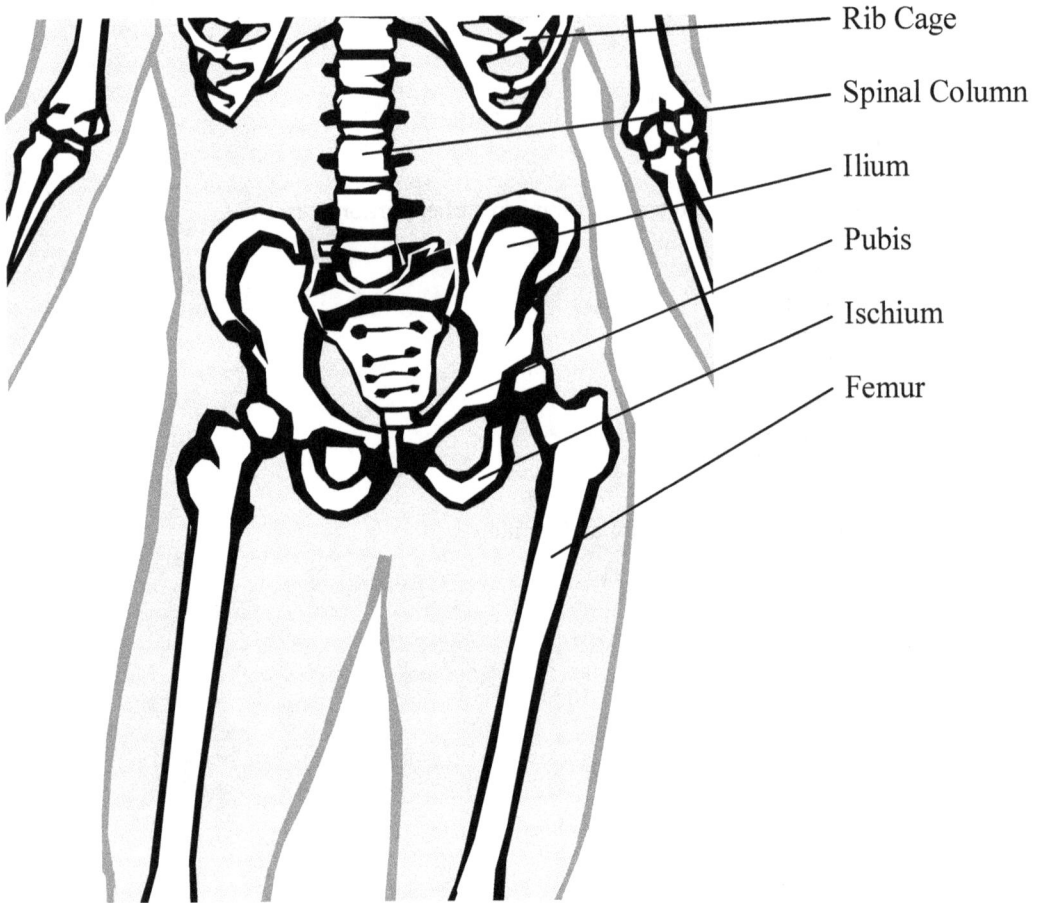

Rib Cage

Spinal Column

Ilium

Pubis

Ischium

Femur

ANATOMY - Muscles

- 650 total muscles in body
- Muscles make up 35% of body
- Skeletal (movement) in 600 directions
- Cardiac (heart)

- Skeletal muscles moved by nerve impulse from brain
- Afferent example; muscles to spinal cord to brain
- Efferent example; brain to spinal cord to muscles
- Voluntary muscles (i.e. skeletal)
- Move only on command from brain
- Involuntary muscles (i.e. cardiac or smooth)
- Function automatically

- When stretching muscles:
    - Warm up muscle first
    - Slow, passive approach
    - Hold stretch 3-5 seconds
    - Don't bounce

- Parts of a typical muscle (see diagram of muscle)
    - Fascia
    - Tendon
    - Bone
    - Periosteum
    - When a muscle contracts shortens thickens widens
    - Synovial fluid helps lubricate muscles, so they slide along side each other
    - Actin (thin)
    - Myosin (thick)

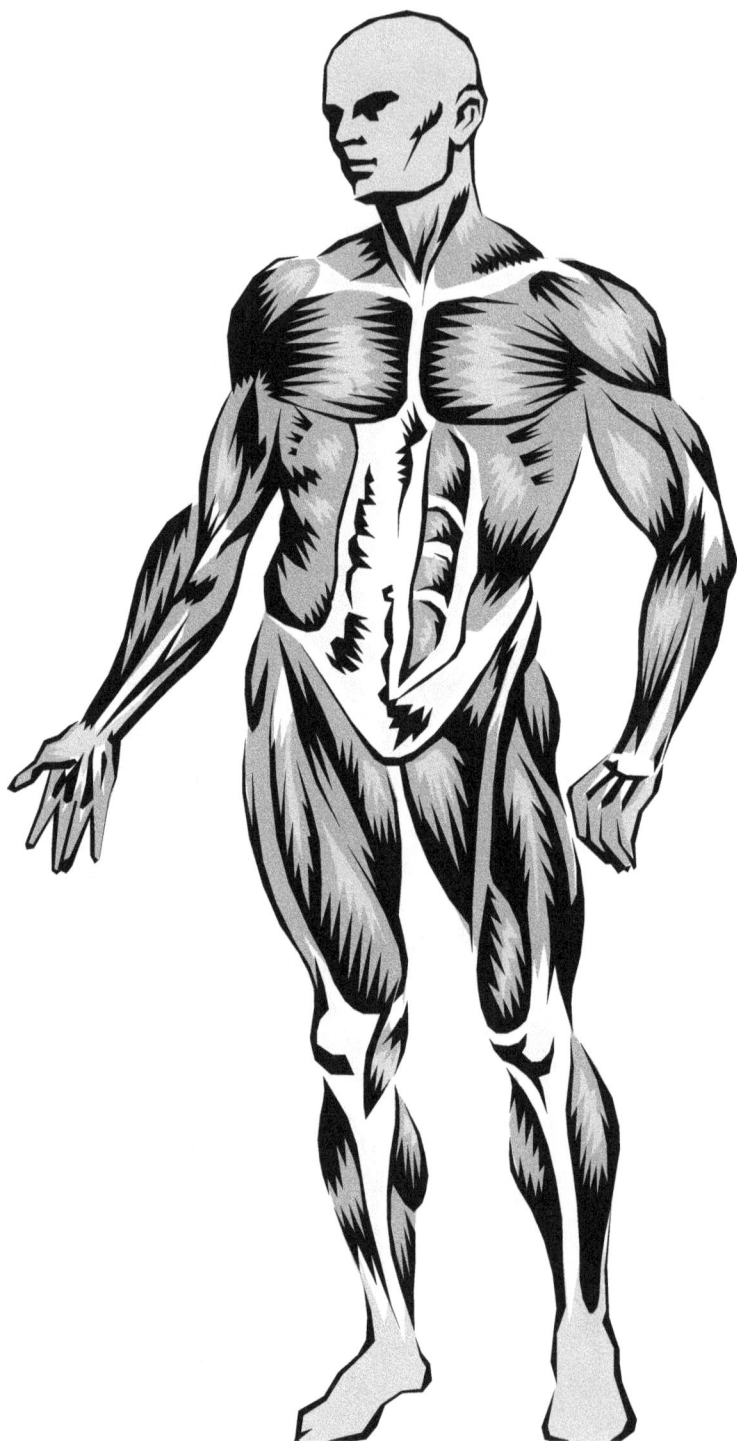

Parallel shaped muscles
- Travel long distance
- Good endurance
- But not real strong
    - (i.e. Sartorius, rectus abdominus)

Fan shaped muscle
- Converge at one point
- Maximum leverage
- Shorter distances
    - (i.e. deltoid pectoralis)

Circular shaped muscle
- Surround an opening
- made for repetition
    - (i.e. oculi (eye) and oris (mouth) muscles

Pennate
- Looks like a feather shape
- Strong
- Dexterity
- Short distances
- Tire quickly
    - (i.e. forearm)

Major muscles to know:
- Neck:
    - Levator scapula
    - Sternocleidomastoid
    - Infrahyoid
    - Suprahyoid
    - Scalene
    - Platysma
    - Splenius capitis
    - Semispinalis capitus
    - Llongissimus capitis

Back:
- Trapezius
- Latissimus dorsi

- Deltoid
- Rhomboids
- Infraspinatus
- Supraspinatus
- Teres
- Serratus
- External oblique
- Erector spinae
- Intercostals

Muscle Shapes

Parallel
- (i.e. Sartourious)
- Travel long distance
- Good on endurance
- Not very strong

Fan
- (i.e. Deltoid)
- For more leverage or
- strength (shoulder)

Circular
- (i.e. Eyes)
- Open and closing qualities
- Repetition

Bipennate
- Very strong
- Distances quickly

Unipennnate
- (i.e. Forearm)

Multipennate
- Dexterity short
- Generally tired
- Bad endurance

- Spinalis (medial)
- Longissimus (intermediate)
- lhocoStahs (Lat.)

Hips:
- Gluteus
- Maximus
- Medius
- Minunius
  - Piriformis (next to gluteus minunius)
  - Iliotibial tract (attached to inferior of gluteus. maximus)

Posterior Legs:
- Semimembranosus (med.)
- Semitendinosus (inter.)
- Bicep Femoris (lat.)
- Hamstring
- Plantaris (post. knee)
- Popliteal (post. knee)
- Gastrocnemius
- Soleus
- Achilles tendon

Arms:
- Bicep, Tricep (17 muscles of forearm)
  - 9 = flexing
  - 8 = extension

Chest and Abdominal:
- Pectoralis major
- Serratus anterior
- Rectus abdominus
- External obliques
- Pectoralis minor
- Subscapularis
- Internal oblique
- Transverse abdominus (deepest)
- Psoas (lower abdominal)

Anterior Legs:
- Rectus femoris (Quadricep)
- Vastus Lateris (Quadricep)
- Vastus Intermedius (Quadricep)
- Vastus Medialis (Quadricep)
- Adductor (Medial of quad)
- Gracilis (Medial of quad)
- Tibialis anterior

Anatomy - Lymph System

- Center of our immune system
- Transports fluids, fat transportation, fights disease

Lymph fluid:
- Slow moving, sticky, white fluid. It is moved along in two ways, skeletal muscle movements and massage. Its job is to return fluids from our body back to the blood. Also it helps protect our bodies from disease, by going through filters called nodes.

Lymph Capillaries:
- Smallest part of lymph system. Very permeable, so interstitial fluid can enter. Lymph fluid (which it is called is now made mostly of blood plasma (low in protein). The fluid has to keep moving (through muscle movement or massage) or edema (fluid caused swelling) will occur.

Lymph ducts:
- Lymph capillaries empty into larger duct system. Walls are similar to veins, they are 3 layers thick. Two main duct systems exist: "Thoracic" (services whole body except right arm, shoulder, and neck); "Right Lymph" (right arm, neck and shoulder area).

Lymph Nodes:
- Small filters which are located along duct systems
- High concentration areas (clusters)
  - Neck
  - Arm pit
  - Digestive tract
  - Groin
  - Posterior part of knee
- 1/3 of all the White Blood Cells are made here, to fight infection and diseases especially types of cancer cells

Lymphoid Organs: (tonsils also)
- These are the spleen (posterior and lateral of stomach) and thymus (anterior of trachea in neck). Spleen helps filter blood. Thymus helps immune system.

Anatomy - Blood and Circulatory System

Red Blood Cells = Red blood cells
White Blood Cells = White Blood Cells

Function
- Its main functions are transporting, immunity, and clotting.

Facts
- Average adult has about 5 liters of blood which makes up 7.7% of the total body weight
- There 60,000 miles of blood vessels that gives life to trillions of cells in the average adult body
- Blood can carry disease-causing viruses, bacteria and toxins.

Arteries:
- Carry blood away from the heart
- Blood is rich in oxygen, because of passing thru lung first, then to the rest of the body.

Veins:
- Carry blood back to the heart.
- The oxygen level is low, because muscles and other cells deplete the oxygen (while they function and do their job)

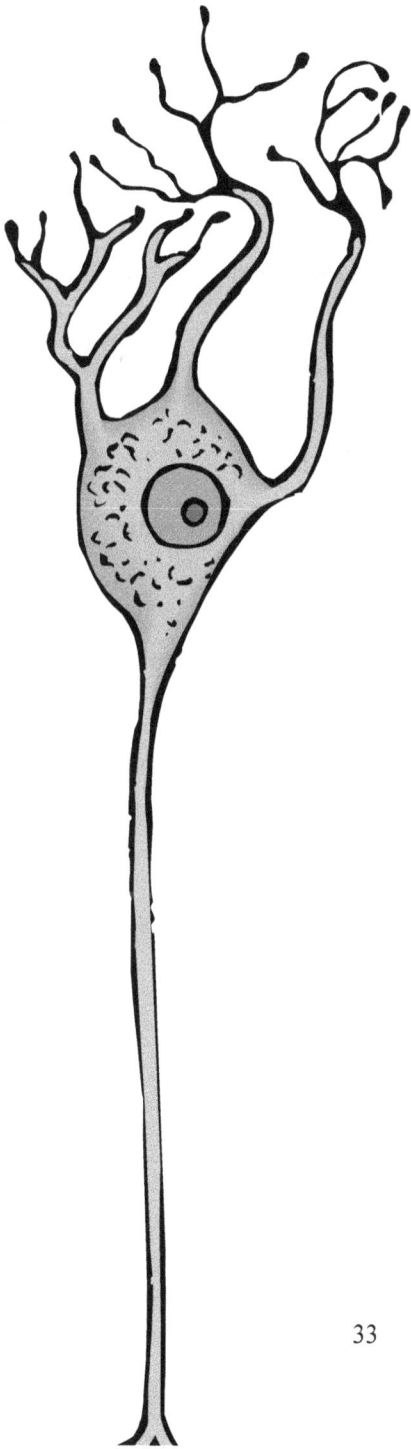

Capillaries:
- Used to connect arteries and veins
- The smallest type of blood vessels thus making a continuous cycle of fluids
- Nutrients and waste are exchanged between veins and arteries thin the capillaries

Interstitial Fluid:
- Fluid that is derived from the clear plasma (blood), that passes thin capillary walls into the surrounding tissue
- Some of this returns to capillaries and some goes into lymph vessels, then is returned to the blood at particular locations in the body

Blood
- Made up of 2 formed elements and plasma
- Red blood cells (RED BLOOD CELLS):
  - (1 cu. millimeter) Most numerous amount in body
- 5.1-5.8 million=males
- 4.3-5.2 million=females
- Flattened and bi-concave shape
- The shape is ideal for carrying oxygen to all tissue cells in the body
- Energy = anaerobic respiration. (non-oxygen fueled organisms)
- Life span 120 days
- Old Red Blood Cells are destroyed by White Blood Cells (also by liver)
- They give blood it's red color
- Rich in protein and iron
- Made in soft tissue inside bones
- Are restricted to veins, arteries and capillaries
- The red iron pigment combines with oxygen in the lung and then to tissue cells all over the body
- Vitamins B 12 and C needed for production
- 2.5 million produced/second

White Blood Cells:
- Life: approx 100-300 days. Some types live only 1-7 days)
- (1 Cu. millimeter) 5,000-9,000 total (male and female)
- 2 types of White Blood Cells
- fight infection and eat waste
- Have a nucleus and move independently
- Can squeeze thru capillary walls
- Are invisible under a microscope
- Most White Blood Cells are made in bones and lymph nodes
- (also liver and spleen)

Platelets:
- Live 5-9 days
  - Smallest of the formed elements
- Actually fragments of larger cells
- No nucleus, but can move independently
- Helps clot blood and constrict vessels
- Old ones are destroyed in spleen and liver

Plasma:
- 55% of total volume of blood
- 90% water, also proteins, salts, acids, vitamins, and hormones
- Purpose is to transport
  - Nutrients
  - Gases
  - Vitamins

Toxins and our body:
- Toxins enter our bodies in many different ways:
  - Air
  - Water
  - Food
  - Medicine
  - Drugs

SWEDISH MASSAGE

History:
- Dr. Peter Ling an Olympic athlete officially developed this style
- Established in early 1800's
- His main interests were in body mechanics, gymnastics, physiology and exercises for women and children
- 1813 the first college offering Swedish massage opened
- The reason the west has been behind eastern massage, was because of the scientific revolution (1700's)
- In the 5th century massage was important to Greek and roman physicians Orientals have been doing their style for 4,000 years

General Facts about Swedish massage:
- Always try to massage towards heart if possible
- Most popular for therapeutic, stress and sports therapy
- 1 hour of Swedish = 5 mile walk to client
- The deeper you go, the slower you go on pressure
- Have your client drink extra water for 48 hours (this helps flush toxins out of body)
- Meditation or centering for therapist makes a better massage It helps therapist stay focused
- Stretches are good to mix in with Swedish
- Infants to elderly need massage
- This is a very universal technique for therapy (it's multi-dimensional)

Four Basic Types of Swedish strokes

Effleurage:
- General, non-specific, gliding strokes
- Basically light pressure
- Warming or to start circulation (this is used also to oil area)
- First step before deeper pressure
- Usually flat, open palm of hand used (spread fingers)

Petrissage:
- A more specific or detailed stroke (medium pressure)
- Pulling, wringing, twisting, stretching, kneading
- Best stroke for increasing circulation
- Work with grain, then do cross fiber, finish with a stretch

Tapotement: (percussion)
- Also known as a percussion stroke
- Medium-deep pressure
- Side of hands, loose fist or cupped hands are best
- Can even loosen congestion in lungs, when done on back

Compression: (deep tissue)
- Deepest of all the strokes
- Remember: This is only done after area is warmed up first
- Elbows, thumb, heel of hand, or forearm used
- Cross fiber technique works well
- Specific areas only

General full Body Sequence
- Oiling (Posterior)
- Neck (Posterior)
- Shoulders/Back (Posterior)
- Gleuts (Posterior)
- Neck/Shoulders (Anterior)
- Upper chest/Abdominal (Anterior)
- Arms/Hands (Anterior)
- Anterior Legs (Anterior)
- Feet (Anterior)
- Connecting Strokes (Anterior)

Full Body Massage Sequence

Neck
- General circular strokes (2-5 minutes)

Back
- Thumbs in-go down spine, return with stretch of skin
- Left Erect-spinous
  - Leap frog
  - Cross fiber
  - Two-hand stretch
- Right Erect-spinous
  - Leap frog
  - Cross fiber
  - Two-hand stretch
- Side pulls (both sides of body)
- Loose fist technique on base of neck
- Double forearm stretch on back (have client take deep breath)
- Metzger zig-zag
- Options: pressure points, tapotement

Buttocks:
- Leap frog/loose fist technique (Option: Pressure Points)

Posterior Legs:
- Leap frog up legs (hamstring)
- 2 hand pettrissage (hamstring)

Popliteal area:
- 2 hand sliding stroke on Gastrocs
- 2 thumb cleaning stroke up through Gastrocs

Scalp and Face:
- Scalp (spider on a mirror technique)
- Various facial strokes

Neck/Shoulders/Upper Chest:
- General circular strokes on neck
- Cervical stretch (pull both hands toward you, rotate hands on edge)
- One hand stretch on each shoulder while other hand provides resistance
- Push down stretch on both shoulders at once

- Clavicle stroke (also thumb strokes between ribs, starting by sternum)

Abdominal:
- 2 hand technique/2 handed plate method (always go clockwise)

Hand and Legs

Anterior Legs:
- Leap frog/pettrissage (quadricep), upward stroke on tibialis anterior
- Opposite with same strokes and sequence

Feet

General Information

How massage therapists can strengthen their bodies:
- Weight training
- Exercise bands, squeeze exercise hand grips
- Squeeze tennis or racquet ball
- Push ups, pull ups
- Yoga classes
- Aerobic exercise classes
- Just doing lots of massages
- Meditation and clear mind prior to massage

Information on Professional Massage Therapy

Typical state requirement for certified massage therapy training:
- Examples
  - California = 100 hours
  - Washington = 500 hours
  - Oregon = 350 hours

Why Therapist Should Start Full Body Massage on Posterior (back) Side of Body:
- Most stress is carried in neck, shoulders, and between shoulder blades
- It's easier to build up the trust of you client. They relax sooner.
- For the beginning therapist it's easier.

General Safety Tips:
- The deep you go on pressure, go slower
- As much as possible work towards heart
- Take your time and get good information from client before starting.

Use Proper Body Mechanics
- Use your body weight for leverage (less wear and tear)
- Good stance (feet and legs) is important
- Use a variety of your body parts as tools
- (thumb, fingers, heel of hand, forearm, elbow)

For profession practic get Liability Insurance ($199/yr. approx)

Proper Draping
- Cover with a sheet or towel for modesty
- Always be professional

Avoid Compromising Situations
- Do not engage in relationships with clients

Always check with clients physician if you have any questions or doubts
- (Even if you have to cancel a pending appointment)

Use a very thorough information sheet to interview your clients - have them respond to the questions below. Here is a sample form:

Massage Client Interview Sheet

- Name_____

- Address_____

- Phone #_____

- Emergency #_____

- Dr. or Physician_____

- Under care of a physician? Yes/No

- Referred by? _____

- Reason for visit_____

- Include a release of liability clause

- Allergies, medications_____

- Record of all massages_____
  _____
  _____
  _____
  _____
  _____

- Signature_____

Potential areas to look for employment:
- Cruise lines/resorts (on the job)
- Sporting events
- Health clubs
- Physical therapy clinics
- Hotels
- Shopping malls
- Community events
- Chiropractic offices

Acupressure (Shiatsu)

History:
- Originally used in China 4,000 years ago
- Came to United States by way of Japan
  - (actively called shiatsu in Japan approx. since 1900)
- Early physicians only had herbs, their hands, and sometimes acupuncture needles for treating their patients (classical oriental blend of medicine and theory)
- Every thing revolves around energy that travels through our bodies, this permitting our body to heal itself (balance or to achieve homeostasis)
- Even modern western medicine has proven that we have energy traveling through specific channels or routes in our body (invisible through the eye)
- Many therapists combine this effective therapy with others
- Swedish, myofascial release, etc.
- Orientals believe everything is divided into two categories or energies.
- Yin and yang. (our body, life and the earth)

Definition
- Means finger tip pressure. Oriental physicians for thousands of years have had success pressing certain specific points on the surface of the body and getting consistent therapeutic results.

Specific situations or ailments: (see diagram of acupressure points)
- Headaches: massage neck, shoulders, upper back
  - Acupressure = Gv15, BL1O, GB2O, 59, B1, St3, Li4, Gv20
- Sciaticia: Put heat on lumbar, sacrum and massage
  - Acupressure = B125, 26, Sacral Notches, Gb30, S74, B136, 37, 57,60
- Lower Back:
  - Put heat on lumbar/sacrum
  - Acupressure = B125, 26, Sacral Nothes, Gb30, S74, B136, 52

- Sinus/Allergies:
  - Put on herbal heat pack on neck and face
  - (Also B120 Th-12) Acupressure: Gv14, Li4, Li20, St3, 6 (C7-TI)
- General Health:
- Acupressure = Li4, St36, Blll, 17; Cv6; LilO (medium fold elbow); T2-3) (T6-7)

Acupressure (Shiatsu)
- Thumb, finger or elbow used to work pressure points on meridians (channels of energy).
- Acupuncture

- Use of needles to work same points (this is not covered in this course)

- Terminology and Information

- Meridians: these are the very important highways or channels that energy travels through the human body.
- 14 total in the body (6 are yin (negative), 6 are yang (positive)
- There are 2 meridians which regulate all of the others
- Governing vesse 1= Yang (positive energy)
- Runs up and down the middle of the back
- Conception vessel = Yin (Negative energy)
- Runs up and down the middle of the front of the body

Yin: (front or anterior side of body)
- Lung
- Spleen
- Kidney
- Heart
- Heart constrictor
- Liver
- Note: each meridian is named for the organ or function connected to its energy flow.
- "Conception vessel" (groin to chin)

- Typical acupressure sure meridian

- Energy circulates throughout the body along a network of passageways called meridians. Traditionally, tsubos are places along the meridians where energy gathers and interchanges between the body arid

45

environment.

- Large intestine
- Stomach
- Small intestine
- Bladder
- Triple heater
- Gall Bladder
- Governing vessel (coccyx to lips)

- Each person can feel the energy move (sometimes it move long distance, sometimes short)
- Pain can be referred long distances also (feet and lumbar) (sometimes pain is influenced by organs)
- Each meridian has pressure points (some have just a few, sometimes many)
- When a part of the body is stretched, the meridian comes closer to the surface of the skin. (so not as much pressure is needed when working each point)
- Since energy flows "one way" in each meridian, if a point is blocked (sickness, stress, etc.), then other points farther down the meridian may be affected.
- I.E. meridians are like canals, energy is like water running through it

- Energy flow stopped
- Excess builds up (tightness and soreness)
- Body is out of balance
- Muscle spasm cycle occurs
- Acupressure breaks cycle, so energy can flow freely again.

- "Pressure Points" (called trigger points or tsubos)
- Three ways to treat pressure points:
- Finger (acupressure)
- Needles (acupuncture)
- Burn herbs on surface of skin (only licensed acupuncture professionals can do this)

- While holding pressure with finger on point, it may take 3 sec. to 45 sec. to release completely.
- Example:
  - 3 seconds = 30% release
  - 30 seconds = 50% release
  - 10 seconds = last 20% release

- 361 pressure points on body
- 92 are used for therapeutic purposes

- Acupressure is used best for preventative maintenance

- If pressure points are sore (stagnant or blocked energy)
- If energy is: Low (deficient has dull pain)
- High (excessive) (has sharp pain

- Pressure point

- Pain = warning signal to our body, something is wrong.
  - (Cancer gives no warning)

- Certain times of day are more effective times to work certain points.
  - (i.e. early morning = lung meridian)

- Working pressure points can increase energy stamina, balance organs so they work at 100%.

- Working an acupressure point
- depth of each tsubo
- Each tsubohas seven layers of energy
- feel sinking to the bottom of the point

Cautions of Doing Acupressure

- Use a safe systematic approach, to each pressure point
- Warm up the area (Swedish massage)
- Apply pressure to point, slowly and smoothly.
- Hold till you feel a full release (remember your thumb may just partially sink into point, not completely) (3 sec.- 45 sec.)
- Ease out of point after release
- Gently massage area and go to next point

- Work abdominal points carefully
- Pregnant women. (Li 4= can sometimes induce labor)
- Also can effect female hormones and release toxins
- Be careful of areas with high concentration of lymph nodes, they could be sensitive.
  - Neck, groin, armpit, etc.
- After acupressure treatment, blood pressure goes down.
- Also recent scar tissue (6 weeks or less)
- Serious burns
- Infections, etc.

"Oriental Philosophy"
- Since the Orientals believe that human body is a microcosm of the universe governed by the 5 elements and the forces of yin and yang.

- Certain elements (and their meridians) can override others. This helps to balance the body. (Example: if kidney meridian is over stimulated, stomach balances)

- We as human beings can accept facts like hot or cold. Sometimes it's hard to accept new things we can't see or understand right away (example the invisible meridians)

Fire
- Active
  - Heart
  - Small Intestine
- 10 a.m.-3 p.m.

Soil
- Downward
  - Stomach.
  - Spleen
  - Pancreas
- 3-7 p.m.

Metal
- Inward
  - Lungs
  - Large Intestine
- 7 p.m. -12 a.m.

Wood
- Rising
  - Liver
  - Gallbladder
- 5 a.m. -10 a.m.

Water
- Floating
  - Kidneys
  - Bladder
- 12 a.m.-5a.m.
- Anatomy wise - what happens in our body.

Introduction to Reflexology

History
- Many people believe it has been around as long as acupuncture (4,000 yrs). It is actually shown in ancient Egyptian drawings from 2,500 B.C. In 1917, an American brought it to the United States. He was physician, and his name was Dr. William H. Fitzgerald. He called it "zone therapy" (10 zones of energy from head to toe on the body) See diagram of foot.

Definition
- Reflexology is based on the principle that there are areas (reflex points), on the hands and feet that correspond to each organ, gland, and structure in the body. A trained reflexologist can accurately diagnose and treat from working points on hands and feet. Average length of a treatment is approximately 30 minutes. Experience determines level of skill.

Benefits
- Most important is relaxation
- Improve circulation
- Better nerve response
- Balance the body and it's systems

Typical approach to working a point

- Warm up the area

- Find the point you desire to treat
- After working the point a few times, leave it for a while
- Return to it, and work it till pain subsides
- It may take a few sessions to get pain to disappear completely.
- Caution: Be careful not to overwork it. (If there is any doubt, refer to a physician.)

Reflexology
Theory and Principles

- As a beginner to reflexology. it is important to study the principles on which die science is based-particularly the zone theory and reflex chztu. These constitute the grammar of reflexology, enabling you to understand how you relax different parts of the body by treating specific reflexes. The zone theory subdivides the body into ten zones, each running through the length of the body. It will help you to familiarize yourself with the theory if you mentally travel up the body from each toe, visualizing the parts of your own body which lie within each zone. The foot guidelines enable you to apply the reflex charts to any shape or size of foot, showing you how to orient yourself with each new partner.

Introduction to Sports Massage

The main, general types of sports massage:

Pre Event
- Light, non-specific, warming. Allows muscles to work more efficiently. Doesn't replace regular warm-ups and stretches. Actually oxygenates muscle cells for maximum performance.

Inter-Event
- Concentration on specific muscles or groups of muscles to be used. Short and light pres sure is most effective.

Post Event
- Promotes relaxation and re-cooperation of muscle potential (oxygen returns to muscle cells more quickly.)
- Reduces muscle tension
- Relieves swelling. Light pressure, general unless you find injuries.

Possible things that could harm the benefits of your massage on client:
- Cramps or spasms = find opposite muscle and contract it (or ice)
- Client didn't train well enough before or prepare correctly.
- Didn't stretch prior
- Imbalance of muscle development (left-right or upper-lower)
- Diet

Swedish is mainly used for sports massage.
- Massage therapists should study, learn, and participate in as many sports for educational purposes. Also reading and studying current techniques and applications of sports massage therapy is critical.

Pre-Event Massage ("Warm-Up")

- Not a substitute for physical warm up or stretching.
- Increase R.O.M. (tense and relax technique).
- Helps muscles work longer and more efficiently.
- Helps athlete have optimum psychic attitude.
- Non-specific, light-med. pressure.

- Basically warming. (15 mm. approx.).

Inter-Event Massage
- Done during breaks, events.
- Short, light pressure (maybe med.).
- Specific, key muscles targeted.

Post-Event Massage
- Promotes a state of relaxation.
- Recuperation time can be cut down (oxygen in muscles helps them to recuperate).
- Tight muscles: tense and relax.
- Ice massage: sprains, cramps, inflammation.

Facts about your body:

- The knee joint is the most complex and largest joint! (see diagram of knee)
- Thickest Muscle = Gluteus
- Longest Muscle = Sartorius

Miscellaneous information about muscles:
- Mother cells that make new muscle tissue cells are called myoblasts.
- Ligaments are for support and protection of joints. They don't heal fast, because they are not very vascular (not much blood goes to them)
- They really hurt when injured, because of the large amount of nerves that go to them

- Levels of muscle strain:
    - Level 1 = partial tear, little loss of function, can hold against resistance.
    - Level 2 = 50% fiber tear, edema, can't hold against resistance.
    - Level 3 = 100% fiber tear, hear a snap at time of injury.

- Note: The sharper the pain, the more severe the injury.

Cryo Therapy
- The therapeutic approach to therapy of injuries using cold (chemical or natural ice)
- Used to treat directly or for re-habilitating process
- In some cases, expedite recovery time by 50%

    Note:
    - 0-48 hours = Cold therapy
    - 48+ hours = Heat or alternate heat and cold (10 minutes each)

- Knee

- The knee is the largest and most complex joint in the body
- Ligaments (Ligaments are different from muscles and tendons)
- Attaches bone to bone-guy wires
- Set limits to our range of motion
- Not as flexible as muscles and tendons
- Doesn't heal quickly because it isn't very vascular

- If Hurt:
    - Ice-constricts veins-desensitizes nerve endings
    - Elevate-keeps swelling down
    - Immobilize-(swelling is body's own way of immobilizing)

5 Ligaments
- On inside medial side of knee is co-lateral ligament
- On lateral side of knee is co-lateral ligament
- Cruciate ligaments

- Patellar ligament

Microtrauma

- Constant repetitive stressing (i.e. Tendinitis) of muscle tissue, leads to microscopic lesions.
- Leads to bleeding and edema. Can result in permanent scar tissue.
- Phases: 1. (Lowest pain) 2.3.4. (Highest pain).

Acute Therapy

- Modify activity.
- Heat before activity.
- Ice and massage after.
- Wear braces and exercise.

Chronic therapy
- Ice before and after.
- Anti-inflammatory drugs.
- Surgery.

Self-perpetuating Inflammation
- Tissue appears to maintain inflammation for long periods of time. (Lasts: months to years)
    - Ice only when muscle is extended

Human reaction to cold therapy (or ice)

Step 1: Appreciation of cold (nerve endings get de-sensitized)
Step 2: Warming sensation
Step 3: Throbbing or aching
Step 4: Numbness

Cautions
- Excess cold therapy = can cause acute frostbite
- Communication with client is essential (leave ice on skin 10 minutes maximum)
- Some people are hypersensitive (only can take a few minutes)
- Wet cold penetrates quicker, follow with R.O.M. stretch.
- Careful where nerves are closes to surface of skin (i.e. elbow, knee, etc)

Cycle of injury
- Ice and massage can break this cycle
- Range of motion stretches and ice can reduce swelling and stiffness
- Massage increases circulation and removes toxins (waste products)

Scar tissue/Adhesions:
- When doing massage we need to think 3 dimensional.
- Petrissage (plucking, griping, twisting, etc.) is best (after approximately 6 weeks of surgery or injury)
- Check with their doctor first, if you're in doubt.

Terminology
- Inflammation = heat, redness, swelling, and fluid
- Contusion = bruise
- Extension of a muscle = narrowing and lengthening of muscle fibers
- Contraction of a muscle = thickening, shortening, widening of muscle fibers
- Mobile scar = scar tissue or adhesion attached to a muscle

- Cycle of Injury

  - Injury

  - Pain

  - Voluntary Splinting

  - Restricted Movement

Example: Carpal tunnel syndrome: Flexor muscles of wrist get overused. Numbing sensation, then pain, stiffness, loss of R.O.M.

Solution: Surgery.

- We can break cycle: Reduce pain with ice and massage.
- We can reduce splinting = R.O.M. + ice
- Increase circulation and detoxify = massage.

Lactic Acid
- Chemical formed by strenuous exercise and accumulates in muscle cells. Only forms when oxygen is depleted in muscle cells.

  - Note: Some lactic acid overflows into blood and lymph ducts. It hampers muscle performance (partial or complete). Lactic acid can go back to original chemical state when oxygen is replaced.

Oxygen shortage
- When our breathing gets more difficult when we exercise. Our body has an O2 debt.

Aerobic
- Exercise using O2

Anaerobic
- Exercise not using O2

Hypoxia
- Decrease of O2 to tissue cells by way of arteries

Hypoxyitis
- Type of inflammation

Hematoma
- Clump of clotted blood, outside vessel

Edema
- Abnormal collection of fluid, under skin

Hemorrhage
- Loss of large amount of blood, in a short time

General muscle information

Fascia
- Fibrous connective tissue that covers bundles of muscle and organ

Main job of muscles
- Movement
- Protection

59

- Insulation

- Oxygen is to muscles, that gas is to an automobile
- Calcium deposits in muscle tissue feels like fine grit or sand to therapist
- Scar tissue or adhesions can restrict range of motion
- Closest attachment of a muscle to the middle of body is referred to as origin. (farthest away = insertion)
- 16 bundles of muscles in forearm
    - 8 = flexing
    - 8 = extension)
- The opposite muscle of a contracting (flexing) muscle is called antagonist.
- The smallest breakdown of muscle fiber (for this class) is actin and myosin.

Lactic Acid
- Pain or burning sensation after a hard work. Comes from "muscle ischemia" (lack of oxygen)
- Pain = stimulating of pain receptors.

Muscular Ischemia
- Produces waste products, lactic acid and potassium which can build up. When to certain point, pain arises.

Delayed Muscle Soreness
- Micro tears in muscle fiber happen because of using muscles that aren't often used. Also from over stretching of connective tissue.

- (Max. Pain)
- (Pain diminishes)
- (Starts exercise)
- + Soreness -
- Misc Sports Massage Information

Common ailments of muscles

Tendonitis
- Overuse of a muscle, gets inflammation.

Fibrositis
- Overuse of a muscle, swelling.

Note: Any time ...it is used, it means inflammation.
Note: Nerve impulse from brain is necessary for muscles to move.

Blood vessels
- Have one way valves also.

Synovial fluid
- Lubricates joints and let bundles of muscle slide against each other.

Digestive System General Notes

Cartilage
- Tough, supportive, connective protects and connects body parts. If tissue in body is very vascular (lots of blood) it heals quickly. If we feel lots of pain from an area, it is highly neural (lots of sensory nerves)

General Anatomy

Stomach
- Expandable, sac like organ. Partly digested food is churned by muscular layers.
- Acids and pepsin enzyme help prepare it for small intestines and further digestion.

Liver
- Largest and one of most complex organs.
- It's found in upper right part of abdominal cavity.
- Weight = 1 lb.
- It detoxifies, regulates blood sugar.
- Eliminates old red blood cells

Thymus
- Located between lungs, near heart Helps children's immune system.

Tonsils
- Help fight infection of ear, nose and throat
- Lymphoid organ (helps lymph system)

Pancreas
- It is about 6 inches long. It is next to stomach.
- Releases a juice to combine with bile to help digestion.
- Also secretes hormones (insulin) into blood.

Kidneys
- Twin organs. Filters wastes from the blood, keeps the Ph balance of the body. Is controlled by hormones, especially from pituitary gland.

Spleen (lymphoid organ)
- Located between stomach and diaphragm in left side of body.
- Part of lymph system. Makes White Blood Cells and destroys old Red Blood Cells and platelets.
- Stores blood and Red Blood Cells before birth.

- Twin elastic, spongy organs.
- Exhales carbon dioxide and brings in oxygen.
- Contain blood vessels, lymph ducts, and air spaces where oxygen/carbon dioxide exchange takes place.
- They inject oxygen into the blood.

Pituitary Gland
- It's attached to hypothalamus control center of brain.
- Helps control certain body functions (body temperature, thirst, and hunger). Divided into two, each has different functions.

Gall Bladder
- It's about 3 inches long. Pear shaped. Located on lower part of liver.
- It is a reservoir for bile, from liver.
- It releases it to digestive tract, to help digestion.

- Many massage therapists keep log sheets to remind and familiarize themselves with clients. Some states have a requirement to maintain these logs. Here is a sample:

Client Log Sheet

Date_____

Name_____

Client_____

Client's Address_____

Clients Phone number_____

Problem or symptom_____

Type of Massage done_____

Total time worked_____

Results_____

Client signature_____

The following pages contain questions to test your knowledge of massage therapy. While these test questions are not meant to prepare you to take any specific examination, they will serve as both a diagnostic and learning tool.

True and False:

1. _____ Your first purchase to start doing massage should be a table.

2. _____ The best area to use for massage is a "bright, well lit" area.

3. _____ If your client doesn't want oil or lotion, use water.

4. _____ A good base oil for massage is almond oil.

5. _____ Most music used by therapists is slow and soothing.

6. _____ Height of table really isn't important

7. _____ The best advertising is "word of mouth".

8. _____ One of the best health benefits of massage is increased

circulation.

9. _____ If a therapist is in doubt about working on someone, see an M.D.

10. _____ The sternum is located in a medial part of body.

11. _____ The occipital ridge is a good place to work for headaches.

12. _____ Eucalyptus is added to base oil to stimulate.

13. _____ There are 650 bones in the body.

14. _____ The stomach filters out toxins in blood.

15. _____ When a muscle contracts, it shortens and thickens.

16. _____ Aromatherapy was first developed by a German in about 1900.

17. _____ Massage therapists can do adjustments of the spine.

18. _____ The cervical section of the neck has 7 vertebrae.

19. _____ Small Intestine (SI 11) is found on the arm (by elbow).

20. _____ When in doubt -whether to massage or not, go ahead and massage/call M.D. later.

21. _____ The zygomatic bone is in pelvis.

22. _____ Patella is the proper name for knee cap.

23. _____ Lungs take in carbon dioxide and put it in the blood.

24. _____ We get vitamin B12 from the sun.

25. _____ Synovial fluid is the lubricant inside joints.

26. _____ The liver is one of the largest organs.

27. _____ Another name for the vertebrae Cl is the atlas.

28. _____ The appendix is very important to digestive tract.

29. _____ Another name for the vertebrae C2, is the atlas

30. _____ Appendix is very important to the digestive tract.

31. _____ The spleen helps digest food.

32. _____ The trachea is for food.

33. _____ The temperature of your massage office is important.

34. _____ Lactic acid is a necessity and a toxin.

35. _____ The closest attachment of a muscle to the middle of the body is the origin.

36. _____ There are 2 layers of gluteus muscles.

37. _____ The lumbar section of vertebrae is part of the tail bone.

38. _____ Lymph nodes make 1/3 of red blood cells for the body.

39. _____ Parallel muscles travel short distances.

40. _____ Oxygen rich blood flows into lungs from the heart.

41. _____ Each bundle of muscle is covered with fascia.

42. _____ The valves inside blood vessels are 2 way.

43. _____ Lymph nodes filter blood.

44. _____ Adult bodies have about 7 liters of blood.

45. _____ Arteries have higher blood pressure than veins.

46. _____ Muscles make up 35-45% of total body weight.

47. _____ Capillaries are used to connect veins and arteries.

48. _____ Swedish massage was established in the 1700's.

49. _____ One hour of Swedish massage=5 mile walk.

50. _____ Tonsils are a lymphoid organ.

"Fill In"

1. Name the vertebrae sections:

    1.1. _____

    1.2. _____

    1.3. _____

1.4. _____

1.5. _____

2. The kidneys filter

    2.1. _____

    2.2. from the_____

3. Acupressure originated from

    3.1. _____

    3.2. about_____ago.

4. If someone doesn't want oil or lotion used on them, you can

    use_____

5. _____is the opposite of posterior

6. _____ is the opposite of superior.

7. Pelvic Girdle

    7.1. _____

    7.2. _____

    7.3. _____

8. Two main types of frames for massage tables are

    8.1. _____

    8.2. _____

9. _____

    equals outgoing

10. _____

    equal incoming.

11. Oriental physicians feel that allows our bodies

    to_____itself.

12. In the stomach

    12.1._____ and

    12.2._____help

       break down food in the stomach.

13. In massage we should work

    13.1._____ the

    13.2._____

14. There are _____ total pressure_____

15. _____is the practice of

    adding _____ extracts to oil.

16. The_____

    is the main part of the immune system.

17. The five elements in oriental medicine are

    17.1._____

    17.2._____

    17.3._____

    17.4._____

17.5. _____

18. Three main types of muscles are

    18.1. _____

    18.2. _____

    18.3. _____

19. Lymph fluid is

    19.1. _____and

    _____

20. Knee joint ligaments

    20.1. 2 = _____

    20.2. 1 = _____

    20.3. 2 = _____

21. _____ is

    what we feel on the vertebrae when massaging the back

Complete the following lists:

What are the health benefits of massage?

1. _____

2. _____

3. _____

4. _____

5. _____

6. _____

7. _____

8. _____

What are the cautions you should look for when giving a massage?

1. _____

2. _____

3. _____

4. _____

5. _____

6. _____

What things should you keep in mind when selecting a massage table?

1. _____

2. _____

3. _____

4. _____

5. _____

6. _____

List 5 possible base oils for massage:

1. _____

2. _____

3. _____

4. _____

5. _____

List 5 possible ways to market and promote yourself:

1. _____

2. _____

3. _____

4. _____

5. _____

List 5 helpful hints for a good massage environment:

1. _____

2. _____

3. _____

4. _____

5. _____

Aroma Therapy: (list the effect of each essential oil)

- Eucalyptus

  _____

- Peppermint

  _____

- Lavender

  _____

- Geranium

  _____

- Camphor

  _____

List 5 bones in the axial skeleton:

1. _____
2. _____
3. _____
4. _____
5. _____

List 8 bones in the appendicular skeleton:

1. _____

2. _____

3. _____

4. _____

5. _____

6. _____

7. _____

8. _____

Identify the part of the knee joint and it's muscles:

1. _____

2. _____

3. _____

4. _____

5. _____

6. _____

7. _____

8. _____

Identify the sections of the skull:

1. _____

2. _____

3. _____

4. _____

5. _____

6. _____

7. _____

Label the muscle shapes:

1. _____

2. _____

3. _____

4. _____

Identify the lymph system:

1. _____

2. _____

3. _____

4. _____

5. _____

List the parts of the spine and the number of vertebrae in each section.

Parts of the spine   Number of vertebrae in each part

1. _____

2. _____

3. _____

4. _____

5. _____

List the order of sequence of the digestive system in the proper sequence:

- Small intestine

- Descending colon

- Ascending colon

- Esophagus

- Rectum

- Mouth

- Stomach

- Transverse colon

1. _____

2. _____

3. _____

4. _____

5. _____

6. _____

7. _____

8. _____

List the cycle of injury:

1. _____

2. _____

3. _____

4. _____

The body (nervous system/acupressure):

1. _____

2. _____

3. _____

4. _____

5. _____

6. _____

7. _____

8. _____

Medical terminology (describe the location in relation to your body):

1. Superior

2. Inferior

3. Anterior

4. Posterior

5. Medial

6. Lateral

7. Interior

8. Lateral

Acupressure: Circuit of change:

1. _____

2. _____

3. _____

4. _____

5. _____

Sports Massage (list facts about each):

Pre-Event:

1. _____

2. _____

3. _____

Inter-Event:

1. _____

2. _____

3. _____

Post-Event:

1. _____

2. _____

3. _____

Pre-Event:

4. _____

5. _____

6. _____

How does a human body respond to cold?

1. _____

2. _____

3. _____

4. _____

Name parts of blood

1. _____

2. _____

3. _____

4. _____

List 5 ways we toxify our body:

1. _____

2. _____

3. _____

4. _____

5. _____

List the muscles that make up the hamstring:

1. _____

2. _____

3. _____

4. _____

5. _____

List the muscles that make up the quadricep:

1. _____

2. _____

3. _____

4. _____

List some facts about effieurage: (a Swedish stroke)

1. _____

2. _____

3. _____

4. _____

5. _____

List some facts about petrissage: (a Swedish stroke)

1. _____

2. _____

3. _____

4. _____

5. _____

List some facts about tapotement: (a Swedish stroke)

1. _____

2. _____

3. _____

4. _____

5. _____

List some facts about compression: (a Swedish stroke)

1. _____

2. _____

3. _____

4. _____

5. _____

List some meridians in each of the following areas: (LI, SI, etc)

1. _____

2. _____

3. _____

4. _____

5. _____

Yin:

1. _____

2. _____

3. _____

4. _____

5. _____

Yang:

1. _____

2. _____

3. _____

4. _____

5. _____

List the areas of body you would massage in a full body sequence:

Posterior

1. _____

2. _____

3. _____

4. _____

5. _____

Anterior

1. _____

2. _____

3. _____

4. _____

5. _____

List the safe sequence to work a pressure point:

1. _____

2. _____

3. _____

4. _____

5. _____

www.ingramcontent.com/pod-product-compliance
Lightning Source LLC
Chambersburg PA
CBHW081701270326
41933CB00017B/3236